The Motivation

Is In You

The Playbook from a Gym Rat

The Motivation Is In You

The Playbook from a Gym Rat

Javon S. White

ISBN: 9798653272325

For information on the content of this book, email blessed_red23@yahoo.com

Cover photo: Shutterstock 52151161

WrightStuf Consulting, LLC
Columbia, SC
www.wrightstuf.com

Printed in the United States of America

Dedication & Acknowledgment

This book is dedicated to anyone who wants to get started on a new journey of being physically fit. It also is for those who might have been on the right path at one point, but somehow seemed to get off track. Just know it can happen at times, and not everyone is able to pick up where they left off. If this is you, I hope this book will give you the push you need to start or either start back again.

To my household family, Quana, Jalen, and Jordan, I am thankful for you all. Not only have you supported my journey, but you are also understanding when you know I need to write about a subject that will help others. To Anita, my god-daughter, my mother, Margaretta, and Lakita, who always lets me know how proud you are of my daily walking during this time, thank you. It helped me to keep going because walking is not my favorite thing to do. To the Quarantine Queens, our coordinator, Dominique, and the other Queens, Veronica, Africa, Asia, Cassandra, and Suzanne, you all have made walking much easier as we walk six days a week. You ladies rock, and I am thankful for the connection even through this time.

Blessings to each person that continues to help me along my journey of life. I do appreciate each person who shows love and support.

To My Facebook and IG followers who are a part of my journey of working out and walking, I appreciate you all, too. There are too many to call out each name, but I do love and appreciate you all. You guys rock, and it is the extra level of pushing I need when you are encouraging me. May God bless each person.

To Toretha Wright with WrightStuf Consulting, LLC, I appreciate all the help you provide for me each time I am trying to complete a writing assignment. You make it easier for me.

Prologue

Spring break 2016 fell in March here in South Carolina. Each spring break, my family tries to go on vacation. This particular year my family went to Florida because they wanted to go to Universal Studios. Well, I am not an amusement park girl. For one, the food is expensive, two, it is hot, and last, I do not ride anything that goes off the ground. I know I am not the only one. But I go because it is to build memories and spend time with the family.

The day we went to Universal Studios was my eye-opener once my Fitbit read that I walked over 18,000 steps. When we walked to the car to go back to the resort after a 12-hour eventful day, I could hardly stand up, let alone continue to walk. I was so sore and exhausted. I know in all my years that was the most I had ever walked in my life. Honestly, it might take me two months to do that many steps. And that moment changed my life for the better.

Instead of looking at my soreness as pain, I looked at it as an opportunity to challenge myself to be a better person. As we got back to our normal life in South Carolina, I told myself that I needed to do better. I had a treadmill and an elliptical at home, and my Fitbit that I had asked for as a Christmas gift and needed to make use of. And guess what I did. The last few days in March was my new beginning of being on the journey to be a better me.

I started at home first before I committed to a gym membership that was not free. So, from the end of March until the end of July, I walked and used the exercise equipment I had at home daily to get me to a place that I would commit to the lifestyle of working out. Guess what? I did it. I did not quit or give up.

July 31, 2016, I joined the gym, and that day I began working towards the goals that I had set for myself. My first goal was losing weight, and because I had a determining mindset, I lost close to 30 pounds in a year. That might not seem significant, but for me, who is not athletic at all, and does not like to sweat, it truly was a big deal. As time passes, I made new goals and began to work on those while maintaining the weight loss.

You determine your outcome, so put in the work so you can see the results!!!!

Contents

Introduction

There is no one size fit all for working out. This book comes from my personal experience that could be a way of encouragement to anyone that wants to get in the game of living a healthier life and being a better you. You are the only one who can determine the outcome, so do not just read this book and go back to or never starting a habit of working out. Allow it to be a help to you.

There are six keys that I found to be helpful for me on my journey. In this book, we will go over those keys. **Determination, Motivation, Investing in you, making time, start moving, and eating habits** have been a blessing to me, and I pray it will bless you as well. I sometimes know we all need a reminder, and I hope this will not only remind you but encourage you.

What made me decide to write on this topic after almost four years on this journey? The new normal of the COVID-19 pandemic gave me some unique insight as the gyms are now closed. What do you do when you cannot go to the place that helps you mentally and physically because the world is now going through a crisis? You still need to do something and not make an excuse.

So, I saw a group of ladies in my neighborhood practicing social distancing while walking through the subdivision. I asked them when and what times do they usually walk. They told me, and I started with them that day. Every day I committed myself to walk at least 10,000 steps or 5 miles whichever comes first, mainly the steps come first. As I write today is my day 28 on this walking journey, and I have walked a total of 417,874 steps/187.3 miles.

How did I do it? Support, determination, commitment, and some good sneakers. And guess what I love the gym, but I hate walking. I could have quit after the second day when my knee started bothering me, but I did not. I ordered me a pair of comfortable walking sneakers and boy does it make a difference. Once my family learned how much I walked, they are cheering for me to keep walking. My son said I could get to 1 million steps by the next few months. I am almost halfway there. I think I can do it. And I will do it

Believe that you, too, can do anything that you put your mind to. I challenge you to put your mind to being better and not only being better but staying better. Let us get to work.

Chapter 1: Determination

When it comes to working out, why is it easier for some to just get it done, and some seem to have excuses? The number one factor is the mindset of determination. What does it mean to be determined? According to Merriam-Webster (2020), it is the act of deciding definitely and firmly; the result of such an act of decision and a firm or fixed intention to achieve a desired end.

How do you decide in all areas of your life? Are your decisions firm or shaky? Do you like results when you accomplish something, or does it matter to you? I want you to say your answers to the questions asked out loud. In fact, read this paragraph out loud. You may be saying, What, Why? I have learned that when we hear ourselves say something out loud, it helps us view the decisions we might make. If it sounds crazy to you, then you will begin to ask yourself why you do some things that way? Some bad habits are learned from generation to generation, and you might be stuck because you thought something was wrong with you. There isn't anything wrong with you if you are willfully trying to do better.

Therefore, it is so important to train our minds to help us reach more promising goals in life. If you do not have order in your life, your mindset will be clouded and less focused. Any bad habit can be reversed only if you want to do your part in helping the process.

This is where you are required to work. Yes, you. I don't believe you decided to purchase this book to let it sit on a shelf. There is something in you that makes you want to have that desire to work out. Buying the book is a great start, but is it not enough to get you to do some form of exercise? In this chapter, I want you to dig deep within yourself and see what is it that might have hindered you in the past to be consistent with your daily routines of working out, if you had one. Or what is blocking you from getting started? In the chapters to come, we will discuss motivation, investing in yourself, making time, start moving, and eating habits. I am sure that made you excited.

To get the best results, you need to learn the real you first. I know, I know, we all want to feel like we don't need help in some areas of our life, but life experiences are not just for us. It truly can help someone else along their journey. We all have strengths and weaknesses. Working out was not one of my strengths before 2016. Then something happened. And I have loved to help encourage and motivate others once I got my routine down.

I believe once you get your routine down and consistent, you will be a blessing to someone else. Now that should help excite you. This is what makes life so much easier to me when we can grow pass our struggles and get stronger to not only help us but help others. Now not everyone is in a place, in the beginning, to help someone else right off the jump, but at some point, in your journey, like myself, you will get there. Right now, just put that in your back pocket, and we can pick that up when you are ready.

Before you go to the next chapter, I want you to do a little homework assignment. Either write it or type it out, so it will be visual to you daily. Write the goals that you would like to start working toward to achieve your best physical health. Do not write outrageous goals in the beginning. Let's first get your mind programmed to take part in your journey.

If you are an analytical thinker like me, let me help you out before you feel like this is not important, or it seems too small. You will add to your list of goals over time, and as you see results, there will always be something else that you want to change. Why do I think this? Well, because we change daily, so in life, we have all learned to make adjustments and adapt to change, even if we do not like it.

Back to why I said do not write outrageous goals. I know when it comes to our physical health, we get frustrated when we do not get the results we had in our minds, and some quit too early. So, when you come up with reasonable and logical results, you feel a lot better. Therefore, our mindset is so important and plays an important role in our level of determination. On the next page, you will find an example of my beginning goals.

I hope it will help you set yours.

Javon's Goals

1. Be consistent
2. Do at least 30-45 minutes of exercise a day/five days a week
3. Lose weight
4. Get off blood pressure medication

Okay, let us talk about this. What did I do to be consistent? First, I started working out at home for four months consistently before I committed to paying for a gym membership that I may not go too. Secondly, losing weight was on my list because I was over my BMI for my age and height, plus when I looked at myself in the mirror, I did not like what I saw. I learned routines that would help me reach my goals. It was a lot of trial and error in the beginning, and I did lose inches before pounds; let me help you out by saying that.

Thirdly, is that I had to take blood pressure medication when I was pregnant. I wanted to be able to stay off medication permanently, so I wanted to do my part in becoming healthier. So, committing to at least 30 minutes a day for five days a week was my start. That might seems like a lot, but I started there so I could push myself in the beginning, go hard and put in the work, and it worked for me. You are not me, and it might not work for you, and that's okay. Your goals might be different, and this is what makes us all unique in our own way.

No matter your goals, even if you think they are small, baby steps are the key to being consistent. So just do what works for you, and please do not compare your journey to others. We are all built differently.

I hope before you start the next chapter, you are more focused and determined to get to a place to achieve results.

You can do it. It is in you!!!

Chapter 2: Motivation

Even the most motivated person needs to be motivated at times. Do you really believe that every person that is working out feels up to it each time they work out? Let me help you by telling you we do not. The difference between each person is what they believe within themselves that they can do it. This is where determination and motivation are important.

As I stated early in the last chapter, I love to encourage others on their journey, so I am very transparent. I do not believe in giving people false truth. My understanding of these helps others out when they are feeling less motivated. The feedback I received from those who followed me on social media helped me out a lot in my beginning stages. It also kept me accountable when I realized that so many people needed my encouragement to motivate them to do something.

It is important that you know all of this because it blessed my life when I shared my testimony with photos of the journey. I received so many comments, even for those who did not work out. People were so impressed with my story; it allowed them to see the results and encouraged them to start somewhere. This will motivate you whether you know it or not.

Honestly, those moments let me know the number of people that really want to healthier. The crazy thing about it, I was not looking for an audience of supporters, but apparently, they were following my journey. How cool is that? Something I was not even good at doing helped me help someone else. I do not know about you, but that made me more determined and motivated.

Before we go any further in this chapter, let us discuss the definition of motivation. Motivation is the act or process of motivating, the condition of being motivated, and a motivating force, stimulus, or influence. Merriam- Webster, 2020.

Think about what or who motivates you. Or it can be both who and what. This can be half the battle of getting it done each time you commit to the process. Getting your mind right is part of it, but doing it is another thing. So, what is it for you? Think. Dig deep.

Let me give you my secret. When I first started, it was not the encouragement I received from others or the feedback because most people, in the beginning, did not know my journey. Even my family around me did not even see how unhealthy and out of shape I was. Only in my 30s, walking in the park of Disney World was a killer that March in 2016. My loved ones just got used to me complaining about how tired I was but never realized that maybe I needed to do something else. The pain I felt from walking persuaded me. That is where it all began.

You might be saying wait. Most people that have pain do not want to add more pain to themselves. Well, the pain made me look in the mirror and realize I needed to do something. That was my motivation.

When I start going to the gym on July 31, 2016, I wanted to cry. I was not athletic at all, and I hated to sweat. To me, that did not equate to anything good in my mind at that time. I did not have the money for a personal trainer, as I am sure they are helpful. But the gym offered a computer program that you can fill in your goals and the results you would like to see so that they can work together with you on a workout routine.

The first day I set foot in the gym, I remember feeling like a dummy. I did not know any of the language for the gym, let alone how to work the machines. When I tell you, I was a beginner, I truly was for the first six months. Like me, if you never had a gym membership, do not let new make you not committed to change. You must try to keep working until things get easier.

Once I got the swing of my plan the computer made for me, I was on a roll, and each day, it was easier and worth the start. About three months in, I had things down pat, and I wasn't as afraid as I was when I first started. The exciting news was I started seeing results.

Did that change the trajectory of my journey? One day I was on the stair stepper, and that was a challenge for me, but every day I got on even if for only five minutes. I wasn't going to be defeated by anything that was a challenge for me. My five minutes turned into 30 over time. Most people were afraid of the stepper. They could last a minute, so five minutes was a big deal.

By the time I made my goal of 30 minutes, one of the personal trainers came to me and said, "Can I apologize?" In my mind, I am thinking, *Apologize for what*? I never paid for a personal trainer, but apparently, my sister had talked to him about tips and pointers, just starting out. She started with me and was more athletic than me, so her form always was more structured than mines.

The trainer had stereotyped me, and he could not hold it; therefore, he wanted to apologize. He said, "I have been watching you since you and your sister started the gym, and I truly did not think you had it in you." He said, "I thought you would have quit before now, but I guess I guessed wrong. And I see you slimming up and toning good."

I smiled and said, "Thank you." I remember riding home that afternoon saying, wow.

Even a stranger doubted me. But that changed the game for me, and it truly built my confidence level to push even when I wanted to give up. As time went on, I kept at it, and more results came. I truly started to feel better. I had lasting energy, and I was feeling good. Who would have ever thought working out could make you feel great and look better? I started celebrating for real after my first anniversary. I had lost 25 pounds. What a difference 25 pounds made for me. I was able to go down from a size 10-12 to a 4-6 during my journey.

Before I started, I was in some 16's and 18's, but I think some of that was because I was insecure about how I looked after my boys were born. I just covered the weight with bigger clothes. I truly feel now my true size was a 14/16. Either way, even if I lost weight and started having healthier reports from the doctor, I was happy. I did it, and so can you.

It was not always easy, but it was worth it. What will it take to motivate you enough to keep going once you start? Is it that new dress, your family, your lab results, or just feeling better about who you are? Sometimes, in the beginning, I had to encourage and motivate myself, but there were little nuggets that helped me continue.

I found a gym family who inspired me and guess what ages they were? They were in their 70's. I watched them do it, and if they could do it, I know I could, so I did and still am even though my gym family is different because of the relocation I made two years ago. But I do have a new family, and we motivate and encourage each other. When we are missing, we look for each other to make sure we keep each other accountable.

If you are new to this, need to get back in the game or start then just tell yourself until you believe that you are worth it and can do anything you put your mind to do. Along the way, there will be help. Just start and do not stop. This is not temporary; this is a lifestyle change that you will be happy you started.

Maintaining is just as important. It is important to remember this nugget as you continue. You do not want to start and see results and get to happy and just feel like that it will stay like that if you do not continue. Never program your mind to think there is an end to this journey. Your goals may change or decrease, and that will be it.

You got this. It is in you!!!!!

Chapter 3: Investing In You

You're worth the investment. Say it with me. I am worth the investment. How much do you believe you are worth? When I hear the word investment, the first thing that comes to my mind is a profit. How about you, what do you think about when you hear the word investment? A gain in profit is always a plus. In the profit of yourself, you will have to put something in to get something out.

Sometimes that is the dilemma we want the profit, but we do not always feel up to putting something in to get it. I do understand, and I am not going to beat you up about it. I have my days and moments, just like everyone else does.

Before we get to a few pointers in this chapter, let me say that each person must do what is best for them and give and do what you can do. If you are an individual that has restrictions due to different health conditions, make sure you, please take the advice of your physician because that is the person who is helping you with your condition. I will just share with you a few of my restrictions and my conditions so it can give you a broader view of my life.

Also, this may be a time that your resources are limiting you to what you can afford to do, but that does not mean you cannot do anything there are so many things available that can benefit us each day. In this chapter, I will share somethings I've learned when life changed for all of us due to COVID-19.

I was a pretty healthy woman in my 20s except for a few migraines here and there. Then somewhere in my mid-20s, I got pregnant with my first child, and life changed. I developed a bad sinus infection during my pregnancy and then pre-eclampsia. The beauty of motherhood, right? But all in all, I was still young. I knew I could get through this and bounce back after my son was born., even if limited to taking medications that were pregnancy-safe. And boy 17 years ago there weren't many choices. I am not sure now, but I am sure it is probably like back then.

After having my first child, 17 months later, I was delivering my second child, still dealing with the effects of pre-eclampsia. Blood pressure became my thorn in my flesh, and I also had allergy issues that caused respiratory problems. Okay, I was learning to deal with it with the help of medication. Then one day, at the age of 34, I developed an inner ear infection that led to vertigo.

I never had an infection in my life before this time. I was walking the track at the park one day, and I told the lady I was with my ear just seemed like sweat kept getting in it, and I was feeling dizzy. So, we stopped and rested for a minute and got back at it. By the time I got home, I felt like I was going to faint, so I had my husband take me to urgent care to see what the problem was.

As the nurse was saying vertigo, I remember saying what in the world and asking why the room is spinning around and around. She smiled and felt terrible for me, as she explained since I was not familiar with her language. I thought okay she will give me something and I will be back to my regular routine in a few days. Ha, boy was I wrong, I was down for a week, and all I could do was go to the bathroom and back to bed, and I needed help to do that.

Why is health so important, and you might be wondering how this might relate to investing in you? Well, if you are limited to what you can do, it will make you feel less of. And sometimes, we do not know there is always an alternative or moderation to what we can do. Because of my vertigo, I am limited to certain levels of exercise, but I do try once to see maybe just maybe it just might not affect me as bad as before.

I will say, over time, things for me have gotten better, and I will tell I think exercising does play a big part in my overall health. I did recently get diagnosed with asthma, but as my doctor figure out the right plan for me, I still will keep believing and pushing to reach my goals rather smaller or big. In my eyes, something is better than nothing.

I try to remain positive and keep hope going so that I do not get discouraged about my conditions. You may have more severe conditions that your limitations are more complex, so again speak with your health care provider and allow them to tell you what you can and cannot do. Once you have a clear understanding, then you will know how to invest in you for the benefit of your physical health.

No matter your limitations, you are so worth the investment. Once you know what you can do, start with that. I know so many people young and old that were on medications, and because they made a commitment to do something, either the medications ended or decreased. I am in that category myself as I write. My physician took me off my blood pressure mediation last year because she said you are healthy, and you work out at least 30 minutes a day, so I think we can take you off.

I was so happy that alone has been a motivation for me not to have to get back on it again. In the first place, I was only on it due to pre-eclampsia during pregnancy. So now, I must focus on cardio, so I can train my heart to be healthier. All this allows me to invest in me, so not only will I be stronger, my health will get better as I put in the work.

Now that we understand how important it is to understand our health conditions and restrictions so we know how and what we can invest in, let us talk about the limitations of resources to be able to work out. Every person does not have the money to afford a gym membership right off. If this is, you know there is still something you can do if that is a limitation for you.

Before I joined the gym in 2016, I walked and used a treadmill that was just taking up space in my house and collecting dust. Also, I had an exercise ball, and elliptical that I would use from time to time. Yes, it was enough to get started. That year I started using the resources I had more than any other year. Finally, I became tired of making excuses. So, I started small before I committed to a gym membership. I knew I would have to pay every month, whether I went or not.

Before this time, I did Weight Watchers for two years, which was a great diet plan that helps program your mindset for the eating aspect of it. I will share that in the last chapter. Even though this was not free, it still was worth the investment. I did reach a lifetime member with Weight Watchers, but time was not on my side then, so I quit. I did learn tools in 2012 that still helps me now. So even if you start something and stop if you develop something else that will benefit you, I consider yourself a winner, nevertheless. So, if you are unable to commit to a gym membership, look up apps that are available online that are free if you have a smartphone.

During this pandemic, the online app has been my best friend since the gyms were closed.

There are so many, and if you do not have a smartphone, walking is free. All you need is some good walking shoes. This is a must.

Walking during this time also is a part of my daily routine. At first, I was not feeling it with my allergies and asthma and a bad knee. Thank God for good working medication, allergy shots, and good walking shoes. Walking seems to be small, but it has some excellent benefits, so never underestimate the power of moving.

If you are able and ready to start working out at a gym, this is fine, too. Whatever is best for you. When you do make the commitment, do not think you have to buy a lot of workout clothes. I started with three appropriate outfits and a pair of sneakers. Old t-shirts were my friend, and still, they are today. Again, I say, do what is best for you.

Check with your employer to see if your company offers gym membership discounts. This can help too. I will say it helped me tremendously. A lot of companies encourage employees to work out. If they are helping, I am getting it.

Whatever way you invest, whether walking, a workout plan, a gym membership, or a home gym, just know you are worth it, and I am so proud of you. You will be happy that you did. I do not regret my commitment; if anything, I regret taking so long to make one. It has been a benefit to my well- being physically, mentally, and emotionally.

I pray and hope you will find a way to do something that can help you in those ways as well. You are worth it. Even if this is the first time you heard, I am proud of you, and I believe in you, I know you can do it. So, let us get it done.

Happy investing in you!!!

Chapter 4: Make Time

Since there are only 24 hours in a day, it seems not to be enough time for us to do the goals we would like to do each day without being overwhelmed. It is easy to get overwhelmed when you have a lot of things to do and not enough time. The average person sleeps and works eight hours a day. That is already 16 hours gone, with only eight to do everything else. And that could vary and not be a full eight hours.

What happens when you must commute to work, cook dinner for you and a family or help a sick loved one. After saying the necessary things out loud, that is already overwhelming. You know what it takes to make things happen in your household, and I want you to start thinking of ways to rearrange your schedule so that you can at least commit to 30 minutes a day for some form of exercising.

What can be eliminated from your day that can help you be more committed and dedicated to your physical well-being? Are you a couch potato, avid social user, gamer, or a talker? You might be one or two or have an issue consuming a lot of your time in these or other areas. Believe it or not, since this is a world of technology, we consume a lot of our time in these areas.

If you are big on technology, use some of your time to commit to an app that allows you to move in some way. Not stay idle. Sometimes it is easier said than done, but I challenge you to try. Trying is better than not doing at all. This part is all up to you and what you can manage.

Time is precious. Once it is gone, you can backtrack time. All you can do is adjust. Keep remembering that you are worth it all. In the beginning, you can always break up your time, if you just cannot manage ding what you need to do all at once.

It does not matter how you work it out just if you do something. Do something when you first wake up for 15 minutes and something else before bed for 15 minutes and that will equate to the 30 minutes for each day. It is possible. Just are you willing to make it happen?

Before the pandemic, I had a balanced schedule that started at 5:30 am Monday - Friday. Each morning I woke up, did my daily devotions, and got ready for the gym between 5:30 and 6:15 am. I would get to the gym right at 6:30 am and stay from that time until 7:15-7:30 am. After I was done, I would go home and shower and get ready for my day from 8:15-5:30 pm.

Morning has always been my schedule because once you finish your workday, most of the time, you are too tired to do anything. So you are not as consistent as you could be if you had more energy. By 8:30 or 9:00 pm, I was ready to call it a night so that I could start all over again the next day.

Now I am an early bird, and I do think mornings are a good time for all my early birds. For my night owls, your time might be better in the evenings after you have gotten settled for the day. Maybe you have someone to help you prepare dinner or do homework if you have school-age kids. Maybe not. Either way, all you need to do is make the adjustments.

Making the adjustment allowed me more energy and a balance in my everyday life. I believe once you put a value on something, you begin to make time for what is important to you. Just like others will spend money on things they want, it is the same with time.

Give it a try and do not make excuses as to why you cannot do something because I am sure you can if you really want to even if you must get your family involved—the more, the merrier. Younger kids are less likely to complain about doing something. If anything, they are more excited and easily trained.

In ending this chapter, my message is this. All you need to do to make time is to prioritize your time. And that might, at times, require you to adjust some things. Challenge yourself. It helps me a lot during basketball season when I get less sleep because of late games with the boys. Make it fun, and it will not seem like a burden or stressful. If anything, it will be worth it when you allow it to work for your benefit.

Chapter 5: Start moving

You must move more than your mind and mouth to see results. If you have already been moving and lose track, get back up and start again. Something is always better than nothing. Since I have been a faithful gym rat since 2016, COVID-19 changed a lot for me this past March. At first, the hours at the gym changed, and the number of people that could enter at one time decreased. Even with the decrease and time change, I was still able to attend three days a week. To me, any time is always better than no time at all. And while I was there, I made it work. I ended up staying an hour and a half compared to my usual 45 minutes to an hour a day. Adjustments are all it takes to make it happen. When the crisis came, one of my first thoughts was what am I going to do about working out. The gym was my outlet, and I had family there outside of my immediate family.

Having a gym family is important. They help keep you accountable when you sometimes slip because of a lack of motivation or other adversity. Some days it will be like that. I just advise you not to stay there. It is always harder to return once you get out of the motion to go and keep going. And that is what I am doing now. I keep going and keep moving.

Walking has become my best friend. I know some might like to walk, but this was not my favorite form of exercising. Don't get me wrong I did it, but it wasn't the first choice. At this present moment, my choices were slim, but hey, so let's work with what we can do. We must stop focusing on what we cannot do. It takes too much of the energy that we need to be committed to a healthier lifestyle.

At the end of March, I tried to get my family on board with this new thing for me called walking. Let me tell you about my family, my two sons, who are teenagers, and my sister, who is younger than me. My sister has a knee injury from college playing basketball, so she is limited to what she can do. If I knew I could depend on anyone, it would be my oldest son since he is an athlete.

The first walk seemed to be going well. It was a nice day outside, not too cold or hot. Might I add we live in the South so if you understand that you know it can get hot? We began our evening stroll. The oldest son and I were walking a little fast, so we turned around and guess what we see? My sister and my youngest sitting down on the sidewalk.

They get back up and attempt to start walking again. The next time we looked, they were nowhere in sight. As we make it home, they are both home chilling. Boy, all I can do is laugh. So, I started thinking, what am I going to do without and walking partners? We live in a big subdivision, but I am not too familiar with the whole area to feel safe to walk alone.

My oldest feels sorry for me and goes with me two days until he sees that I am walking more than I did the first day. He quits on me, as I was just getting on a roll. I prayed and said, Lord, let me find someone that I can walk with that walks as fast as me who will not quit.

The Lord knew what I needed because walking was not for me at all. I did not need anyone to motivate normally for working out. I just did it.

But I needed some help with the walking thing. Walking can be kind of boring when you are alone. But I needed to do it even if I had to go alone. Then one day, I was looking out my window, and I noticed people walking on my street.

The people I saw that day I remember I had seen them a few days ago when I was hanging outside. I spoke to them, and they returned pleasant greetings. The next time I saw, me being friendly, I go to my porch and say hey to them and ask if they walked every day and what time. The lady who started the walking group said yes, we do, and we are walking in the morning and evening. I said okay I would like to start walking with you tonight and then start in the morning.

I knew the evening was not my thing, but I started that day because if I did not, I would have had too much time to talk myself out of starting this new process. And then, tomorrow, I transitioned to my regular programmed schedule of mornings.

I realize most people like to wait until they feel like it or the new year to say they will commit, some right start off they strong for that first month because the excitement is good, and it seems right then. What happens when it is not so exciting?

Normally you quit. I advise if you are going to do something to help you, health-wise, do not wait. The moment you think about it, start then.

I joined the gym on July 31, 2016. That was no special day, but it became my anniversary date once I reached my year. Trust me, you will remember the date just like yesterday, no matter when you start.

Today is day 42 of consistently walking every day. To make it challenging for me, I committed myself to at least 10,000 steps or 5 miles a day. It did not matter what the group that I asked to join was doing, this was my personal goal. And guess what? I have been doing it each day. I have walked a total of 610,169 steps/280 miles. And today, for the first time in about 20 years, I ran 1.5 miles without having to use my asthma pump. If you just try, you can do anything you put your mind to.

I am really starting to enjoy walking. I know I am getting good vitamin D now because before it was deficient and I had to take a supplement. So even when you feel like things do not work out, it will, if you will remain positive about the outcome.

I am thankful that I prayed to God about the support for me during this time. Our coordinator has encouraged others to join us, and there are at least five of us that consistently walk while practicing social distancing. We all walk at our own pace, and it helps during this time that we are not so close to each other.

Our walking ministry is called the Quarantine Queens, and we promote so much positivity to each other. It has been all worth it. I love to encourage, and it has been so rewarding even if they were strangers that now I can grow to know. My kids thought I was weird to just ask to be included, but I am a friendly person, so this was right up my alley.

The group pushes each other, and we celebrate each other. One of the ladies had a doctor's appointment today, and her doctor told her that he was pleased with her. He asked her what she was doing for the last two months because she had lost 10 pounds. She said, "I joined the walking ministry group." He told her to keep it up.

Once everyone's schedule changes, we will have to adjust, but once you start something, it's hard to just quit when you start seeing the results. You will make the adjustment. Remember, you are worth it. Because of them, I decided to write this book. I always loved to support, encourage, and motivate. One day as I was walking, I could hear the Lord saying, *write, you can help so many*, and here goes I hope this will help you.

You might not have a success story like me. Maybe you can be the coordinator. Don't wait for someone else to do it. Be the one to make it happen. I used to hear a quote, "Excuses are good for the ones giving it." So, before we move on to the next chapter, what is your excuse? Maybe you don't have an excuse. Either way, suck it up, and let's get moving. You can do it. It is in you!!!!

Chapter 6: Eating Habits

I know this is not the easiest chapter to write, but this book would not be complete unless I gave you all that I have learned on this journey. When I first started going to the gym, my number one focus than was determination and consistency. Food was not on the top of my list. So, you might be wondering then why are we talking about it? Trust me, there is a reason.

I am by no means a nutritionist or expert, but I have learned that there is a method to the madness. I learned before my beginning stage of working out from the weight watchers' program in 2012 that you can eat certain things and lose weight. Back then, they used to give you a certain number of points you could eat a day depending on your weight, sex, height, and age, I believe. If you would stay in your range, you would at least lose 1 pound a week.

Do not give me the side-eye when I say one-pound average a week. You are like really; I must do all this to lose one pound? One pound is a healthy place to be if you are trying to lose weight and keep it off. Sometimes we try to do it the unhealthy way and lose too much at one time and gain it all back quickly. They call that yo-yo dieting, which is not good for your body or your metabolism.

For me personally, it has been easier for me to maintain my goal weight when it took me longer to get there than getting there faster. I do not believe in the word diet at all. Diets, to me, set people up for failure unless it is a sustainable plan that is healthy and will be a lifestyle change and not a diet. Save yourself the stress.

All we need to do is pick better food choices and eat foods that will fill our body and give us the nutrition that we need. When I eat the proper foods, I feel better, and I even look better. I know it seems it costs a lot to eat healthy. Sometimes it does, but sometimes just adjusting what you eat can make a difference in your body.

Why did I mention weight watchers? I truly enjoyed and learned something from this program. You could eat whatever you liked, but you just had to know how many points it would cost you from your daily food count. There were a lot of foods that were 0 - 2 points, and can you guess which foods they were? If you guessed fruits and vegetables, you are correct. This program made me more aware of what I was eating and helped me be more accountable.

Even though I do not attend the meetings anymore, and I am sure they have revamped the program, it still influences the choices I make in my eating habits. Not to say that I always pick the healthier choices, but I do try more than not.

A typical food list for myself is as follows. Fruits, beans, vegetables, smoothies, salads, fish, chicken, shrimp, pork, and beef. And I need to be honest, I have a small home-based business called "A Taste of Love, LLC." So, I do bake, and I love sweets. Sweets is where I go wrong.

We all have an issue with some foods. Yours could be bread, carbs, or sodas. Whatever it may be, I advise you to try to do things in moderation so that you do not feel deprived. People give up because making better choices sometimes feels like a punishment. Making some adjustments will help you become more committed to your journey.

Do not let me forget to encourage you to drink, drink, and drink your water. This is good for you. Water will help your process and it is essential to our well-being. If you do not drink water now, start and keep doing it. I try to drink 6-8 cups of water a day. The days I don't drink water, I don't feel as energetic as when I do get my daily intake. It does make a difference. Add water and other healthy beverage choices that will help you to your everyday routine.

Kid's meals are a part of my eating habits when we do not eat at home. This helped me to program my stomach for smaller portions of food. If you don't want to eat a kid's meal, then try eating smaller portions. Sometimes, a big plate of food will make you feel like you have to eat everything on the plate at one time.

Each day we all must make a choice to do things that will benefit us, not just now, but in the future. Do not try to stop all the bad habits cold turkey. Do each step-in moderation. It is all in you. You can do it. Believe you can and you will.

Conclusion

You will always be your number one fan. You can do anything you put your mind too. Positivity can take you a long way. Remain positive during this journey. Do not be negative about where you might be. Whether you need to lose a few pounds, get a better routine, or tone up, it does not matter you can do it. Surround yourself with people that will motivate you and support your journey. Remember, this is not temporary; this is a lifestyle. Your life is in your hands, and you hold the key to your success.

Look in the mirror and envision yourself where you would like to be. Nothing is too big or too small. Every goal you make will be an investment in you. You are worth it all. Be determined, dedicated, and consistent with your process and your outcome.

Do not compare yourself to others. Everything that you see is not the whole story. Write your own story and know that someone needs your motivation to help them. Yes, one day, you will be able to help someone else. It will always be so worth it in the end. You can do it. Let us get moving. Be consistent, adjust, eat the best you can, and do not quit.

Happy moving!!!!

Meet the Author

Ms. White is a woman of God who believes that with God, all things are possible if we just believe. She truly gets excited when she thinks of the Goodness of Jesus. Ms. White is blessed to be called mom to two wonderful teenage boys, Jalen and Jordan. She also has a Goddaughter named Anita. Ms. White is blessed with some wonderful people in her life who she calls family. Her bonus sister Shaquana and deceased spiritual Mother Carolyn are the two who pushed her to write and to continue to write.

Ms. White is thankful for all the support of her loved ones because, without their support, prayers, and love, she would not be able to effectively walk in this level of purpose.

In her free time, she takes heart in praying for others. She loves the babies she keeps daily and takes heart in being a part of their life. When she is not caring for others, she loved to go to the gym, shop, basketball games, cook, and be creative with arts and crafts. As you read this book, she wants you to feel the prayers she is praying for you and your family.

Read other books by the author

Seeds of hope

Walking in Purpose

How relationships shape who we become

Living a Holy and satisfied life single

Draw near to God